DIY Placenta Edibles: Smoothies + Tinctures + Chocolates

By Katie DiBenedetto

Acknowledgements

Special thanks to Nancy, who trusted me with her placenta (my first one!) even though I didn't know what I was doing. To Kewal, who instructed me how to prepare Nancy's placenta. To Danielle, my partner in learning for those first few placentas. And to Shell Walker, who started the Placenta Liberation Front (just one of many of her brilliant ventures), which provides an incredibly thorough and completely complimentary training on placenta prep, the only requirement being that you obtain all of the necessary supplies for professionalism and safety, that you go forward and teach other people, and provide your first few placenta preparations for free. I have learned so much from Shell and am grateful that my path has crossed hers in this life.

Table of Contents

Preface

I wrote this guide for women. For women who perhaps aren't surrounded by other womenfolk who are full of knowledge and wisdom. For women who are curious. For women who want to know. For women knowing they want to do something with their placenta, but aren't quite sure what to do. For women who want somewhere to start, some steps to follow, some photos to help them along. I hope you find what you are looking for here ☺

Placenta crafting is not and should not be a "secret" that is guarded by "professionals". It is an act of love and gratitude that takes nothing more than a pair of capable hands and a few simple tools.

I am honored anytime a woman trusts me with the preparation of her placenta. Though I am delighted that it is one of the ways I sustain myself, I would never hesitate to empower a woman with the same knowledge and skills that I learned from my women friends and teachers. The wisdom that I hope you will pass on to your daughters, your friends and your sisters.

From my heart to yours,

Katie

Feel free to contact me with any questions that come up!
Katie@2doulasonamission.com

Placenta Benefits

The benefits of consuming your placenta are endless! Did you know that, other than camels, humans are the only mammal that doesn't consume their placenta?

First and foremost, the placenta is an organ, so it is chock full of iron & other nutrients. On top of that – your placenta is full of hormones, which help balance your system after birth.

Placenta benefits:

- Contains your own natural hormones

- Is perfectly made by you, for you

- Balances your system, replenishes depleted iron

- Gives you more energy, lessens postpartum bleeding

- Has been shown to increase milk production

- Helps you to have a happier postpartum period by equalizing the quickly reduced hormonal state of your physical body

- Helps to hasten the return of your uterus to its pre-pregnancy state through the oxytocin contained in your encapsulated placenta.

- Can also be helpful during your monthly cycle, menopause, for general mood swings, periods of major life transition, etc. if properly stored for later use.

- Visit our website - 2doulasonamission.com - for other articles & info about placentas.

Safety & Sanitation

As stated in the opening disclaimer (which is a bit harsh but, you know, necessary in this big world) this guide is not intended for use by anyone other than the individual woman (and her trusted family and friends) preparing her own placenta in her own home with her own equipment. May I reiterate that this is not at all the appropriate way to learn about placenta preparation if you are intending to have a placenta business and prepare the placentas of women that you don't know. If you are inspired to offer it as a service to your community – thank you! We need more women like you! Just please make sure you are properly trained and learn the necessary safety procedures with regards to sanitation, blood borne pathogens, etc.

As I'm sure you know, placentas are messy. It would be wise to clear yourself an area – a countertop, a table, somewhere that will minimize blood drips and splatters, simply for easier clean up. Make sure your area is large enough that you can have all of your supplies near you so you're not walking back and forth or scattered.

When you work with your placenta, be sure you are present and inspired. Put on your favorite music. Take a moment to thank your placenta and recognize what an amazing gift it gave to you and your baby. Try to keep your mind clear and your thoughts positive so as not to infuse your placenta with anything other than peaceful, joyful intentions and energy.

Supplies List + Where to Buy

Please note – this is not a list of everything you need to go out and buy. Some supplies are optional, some supplies overlap, and some supplies you only need for a specific method. This list is simply to act as a reference guide for definitions of different supplies, where to get them, what not to use, and so on. A simplified, bullet pointed supply list is listed with each method of encapsulation. Please make sure you read over this descriptive supplies list, decide what encapsulation method you want to use, and read through the instructions before you decide which supplies to get.

Scissors or a knife: I use stainless steel scissors that come completely apart. You can find these in the kitchen section of most stores. They're easy to clean and easily cut through the placenta. You could also use a knife – make sure it is very sharp. I would recommend partially freezing the placenta so that it is more solid and easier to slice with a knife.

Gloves: optional. Non-latex disposable gloves are best – the kind a doctor or nurse would use when doing an exam. I buy mine at Costco. Do not use plastic food prep gloves.

"Tray": this could be a cookie sheet, a tray, a cutting board or any other flat surface to place the placenta on while you're cutting it up. If you are using the raw method, it's helpful if your tray has a lip to aid in catching drips and keeping the blood contained. With the TCM Method you will have drained the placenta of blood so having a lip on your tray is not necessary.

Dark glass one-ounce bottle with lid: You can find these at Whole Foods, at most vitamin or herb shops, or online, or reuse one that you already have.

Dark glass one-ounce bottle with dropper: You can find these at Whole Foods, at most vitamin or herb shops, or online, or reuse one that you already have.

Alcohol: I prefer 100+ proof Everclear, but you can also use brandy, vodka, or whiskey.

Cheesecloth + rubber band: If you don't have cheese cloth, any sort of meshy, breathable fabric will do. You want to keep dust and debris out, while still allowing air to flow. You will use the rubber band (or piece of string, twine, etc.) to secure the cloth around the lid of your tincture while it's curing.

Distilled or spring water: spring water is ideal, but if you don't have a spring near you, distilled water will do just fine.

Placenta powder: dehydrate and powder your placenta in the way of your choosing. If you need instruction, you can find that in our first book in this series "DIY Placenta Encapsulation: A Step-by-Step Guide".

Double boiler: this can simply be one medium sized pot sitting on top of a small sized pot.

Candy mold: you can get these at most craft stores or cake decorating stores.

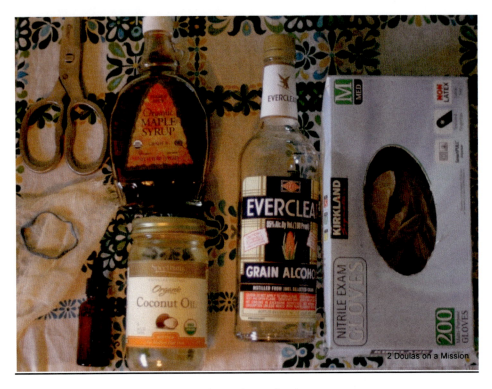

{A sampling of supplies}

Placenta Tincture

Supplies:

- Scissors
- Gloves, optional
- Tray
- Small jar
- 1 ounce dark glass bottle with lid
- 1 ounce dark glass bottle with dropper
- Alcohol
- Water
- Cheesecloth
- Rubber band

Instructions, Part One: Making the mother tincture

- Put your gloves on, if using.
- Place your placenta on a tray.
- See where you feel called to remove a piece of your placenta. Using your scissors, you can remove a chunk from one particular spot, or you can remove several smaller pieces from different spots such as the maternal side, the fetal side, the cord insertion point, etc.
- The size of the piece is entirely up to you. Generally, a piece or pieces totaling the size of a half dollar coin is used. You can make quite a bit of tincture from a small piece of placenta.
- Once you have removed your piece(s), place them in your small jar.
- With the placenta piece(s) in the bottom of the jar, pour alcohol into the jar until you reach a level an inch or so above the placenta pieces.
- Cut a piece of cheesecloth to fit over the top of your jar.
- Secure it to the mouth of your jar with a rubber band.
- This will be your mother tincture. You may want to label and date it for your reference.

- Place your mother tincture in a cool, dark place to cure. If you feel called to put your mother tincture in the sunlight, or under the light of the moon, by all means – do it!

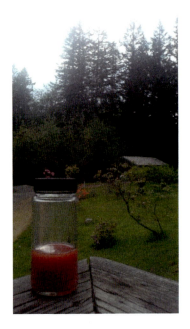

{Mother tincture curing on a sunny balcony}

- The length of time is up to you and you will just have to feel it out. It can cure anywhere from 3 days to 6 weeks or longer. You'll want to check your tincture every few days to replace any alcohol that may have evaporated.

Instructions, Part Two: Getting your tincture ready to drink

- Once you feel your mother tincture is done curing, strain the liquid through the cheese cloth and into your 1 ounce bottle with lid. This is now your mother tincture.
- You may wish to bury the pieces of placenta that you used for your tincture.
- Into your glass bottle with the dropper, put 30 drops of your mother tincture, followed by alcohol until you reach the half way mark, and water until you reach the top (leaving head space for the dropper).
- You now have a ready to drink placenta tincture!
- You may continue refilling your placenta tincture dropper bottle as described above.
- Every few times you refill, top of your mother tincture bottle with more alcohol so that you can keep making tincture for many years to come.

Placenta Smoothie

You can use any smoothie recipe that you'd like. For the sake of simplicity, I'll list ingredients for the most popular one I've come across.

Supplies:

- 1 cup fresh squeezed organic orange juice
- ½ cup plain organic whole-milk yogurt
- 1 cup frozen strawberries
- Scissors
- Gloves, optional
- Tray
- Half dollar size piece of fresh placenta

Instructions:

- Put on gloves if using
- Place your placenta on a tray and
- See where you feel called to remove a piece of your placenta. Using your scissors, you can remove a chunk from one particular spot, or you can remove several smaller pieces from different spots such as the maternal side, the fetal side, the cord insertion point, etc.
- Place placenta pieces along with ½ of orange juice into your blender.
- Blend on high for 1-2 minutes.
- Add remaining orange juice, yogurt and strawberries.
- Blend on high until well incorporated.
- Serve in a gorgeous glass with a colorful bendy straw.

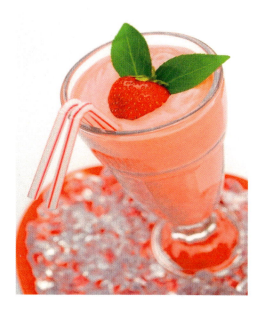

Note: if smoothie is mamas preferred way of consuming her placenta, then you may want to go ahead and cut up the entire placenta into smoothie sized pieces. Place the pieces in a single layer on a cookie sheet lined with parchment paper and place in the freezer. Once completely frozen, you can put the pieces in a jar or other storage container and keep them in the freezer.

Placenta Chocolates

- Your placenta powder
- Coffee grinder
- Fine mesh strainer
- Large bowl
- 1 pound high quality organic dark chocolate
- Large knife
- Cayenne pepper
- Cinnamon
- Double boiler set up
- Spoon
- Candy mold

Note: *This recipe is based on the amount of placenta powder from an entire placenta. If you are only using part of your placenta for chocolates, then adjust the amount of chocolate accordingly.*

Instructions:

- If you originally ground your placenta in a coffee grinder and it is already very fine, then you can skip this next step.
- Grind your placenta powder in a coffee grinder until it is very fine – you may need to do it in several batches.
- Place your fine mesh strainer over your large bowl and strain your placenta powder into the bowl. The strainer will catch the bigger bits of placenta that would be unpleasant to have in your chocolates.
- Bury the bigger bits, or pop them into capsules and consume them.
- Set up your double boiler on the stove and begin melting your chocolate.
- Roughly chop your chocolate
- Begin melting chocolate chunks in your double boiler

- Once your chocolate is melted, add your placenta powder and mix until incorporated.
- Using your spoon, begin filling your chocolate molds.
- Place mold in the freezer until chocolate is set, about 15 minutes or so.
- Pop out your finished chocolates and repeat until you have used all of your chocolate mixture.
- Store your finished chocolates in a container in a cool, dark place – often the fridge is the best spot.

- **Note**: *If using a standard bite sized chocolate mold, 3 chocolates typically contain the same amount of placenta powder as one capsule would.*

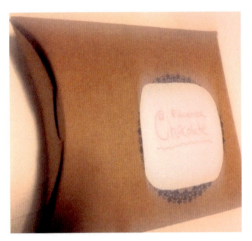

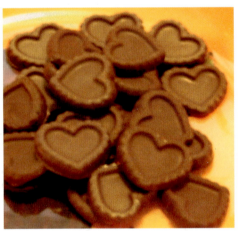

Placenta Truffles

Ingredients:

- Placenta powder
- Coffee grinder
- Mesh strainer
- Large bowl
- spoon
- ½ cup unrefined, organic coconut oil
- ¾ cup organic coconut butter
- 5-6 tbsp raw cacao powder
- 2-3 tbsp maple syrup
- Sea salt to taste
- Double boiler set up
- "peanut butter cup" style candy wrappers

Note: *This recipe is based on the amount of placenta powder from an entire placenta. If you are only using part of your placenta for truffles, then adjust the ingredients accordingly.*

Instructions:

- If you originally ground your placenta in a coffee grinder and it is already very fine, then you can skip this next step.
- Grind your placenta powder in a coffee grinder until it is very fine – you may need to do it in several batches.
- Place your fine mesh strainer over your large bowl and strain your placenta powder into the bowl. The strainer will catch the bigger bits of placenta that would be unpleasant to have in your truffles.
- Bury the bigger bits, or pop them into capsules and consume them that way.
- Set up your double boiler on the stove and begin melting the coconut oil and coconut butter.
- Add your placenta powder and mix until incorporated.

- Add the cacao powder, maple syrup and sea salt until it tastes good to you. Some people like more salt, less syrup, more chocolate, etc.
- Mix until incorporated.
- Set up your candy wrappers on a tray
- Using your spoon, fill your candy wrappers half way with your truffle mix
- Place tray of truffles in the freezer until set, about 15 minutes or so.
- Store your finished truffles in a container in the fridge or freezer.

Note: each truffle generally contains the same amount of placenta powder that one capsule would.

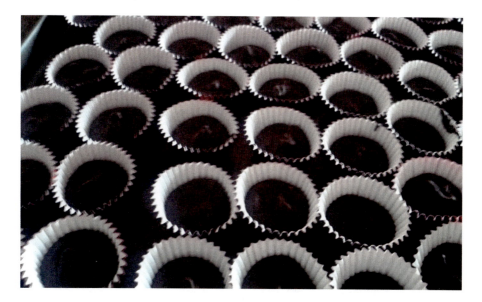

Dosage

Your placenta may be shared with anyone that you wish. Often times families enjoy consuming the placenta together with mom, dad and older siblings partaking. Tincture can be a great way to share placenta with baby and use as a remedy during teething, growth spurts and bouts of fussiness.

Chocolate or smoothies is a favorite way to share the placenta with the child as he/she gets older.

I would be making it up if I told you a dosage – anyone would. Each placenta is different in size, weight and overall composition. Each woman's need are different. Some women take their placenta with food, some don't. Some don't consume it too late in the day as it gives them too much energy, others don't feel this at all. Dosage is completely self regulated and you'll just have to play around with it. If you have a specific goal in mind – a higher milk supply, less mood swings, etc. then take more. If you're having an especially bad day – maybe take a few more than you would on a good day. Once you find your sweet spot – stay there for a week or so and then gradually take a bit less and see what happens.

General dosage starting points:

Tincture: Adults – 30 drops at a time, children 15 drops, babies 5 drops – may put in milk or juice to help mask the strong flavor from the alcohol.

Chocolates: Mama: 3 pieces twice per day. On an as needed basis for anyone else.

Truffles: 1 piece twice per day. On an as needed basis for anyone else.

Other Placenta Uses

There are certainly many more things you can do with your placenta besides what's listed in this book. First and foremost: you can encapsulate it. As mentioned earlier, our first book shows you how to do just that: "DIY Placenta Encapsulation: A Step-By-Step-Guide".

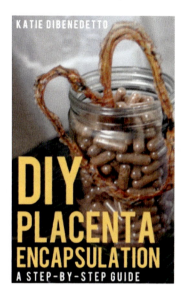

Additionally, you could get crafty with it. Make a few placenta prints, take some photographs and preserve the amniotic sac. Instructions on making those delights can be found in "DIY Placenta Art: Prints + Photos + Cord Keepsakes"

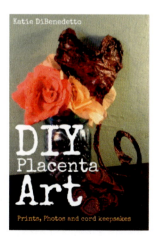

You could also plant the placenta or part of it in a spot significant to your family. You could even plant it in a pot so you can take it with you always.

You could prepare the placenta as you would most other pieces of meat: grill it, put it in chili or a lasagna, make a yummy stew, etc.

Get creative! Have fun!

Resources

DIY Placenta Encapsulation: A Step-By-Step-By-Step Guide" available on Amazon in e-book or hard copy format. Instructions for the Raw Method or the TCM Method of encapsulation.

"DIY Placenta Edibles: Smoothies, Chocolates, and More!" available on Amazon in e-book or hard copy format. Instructions for making various edible options.

DIY Placenta Art + Encapsulation: my facebook page where I post updates, photos, ideas and other placenta related things.

2doulasonamission.com: my website for blogging, e-books, doula services, placenta crafting and other forms of birth art. You can also find my contact info here. Feel free to reach out if you have any questions!

Placenta: The Forgotten Chakra, by Robin Lim (http://gaia-d.com/robin-lim-e-books/)

Placenta: The Gift of Life, by Cornelia Enning (http://www.midwiferytoday.com/books/placenta.asp)

The Amazing Placenta, by Sarah Buckley, M.D. (http://www.mothering.com/community/a/the-amazing-placenta)

The Amazing Placenta, by Suzanne Nguyen (http://m.theatlantic.com/health/archive/2013/12/the-amazing-placenta/282280/)

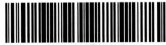

Made in the USA
Middletown, DE
13 July 2018